THE HEALTH BENEFITS OF MEDICINAL MUSHROOMS

Mark Stengler, N.D.

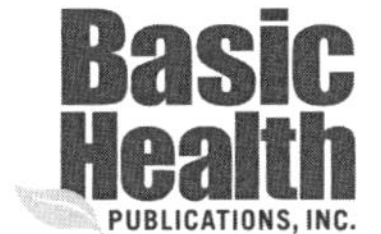

The information contained in this book is based upon the research and personal and professional experiences of the author. It is not intended as a substitute for consulting with your physician or other healthcare provider. Any attempt to diagnose and treat an illness should be done under the direction of a healthcare professional.

The publisher does not advocate the use of any particular healthcare protocol but believes the information in this book should be available to the public. The publisher and author are not responsible for any adverse effects or consequences resulting from the use of the suggestions, preparations, or procedures discussed in this book. Should the reader have any questions concerning the appropriateness of any procedures or preparation mentioned, the author and the publisher strongly suggest consulting a professional healthcare advisor.

Editor: Carol Rosenberg
Typesetter: Gary A. Rosenberg
Cover Designer: Mike Stromberg

Basic Health Guides are published by
Basic Health Publications, Inc.
8200 Boulevard East
North Bergen, NJ 07047
1-800-575-8890

ISBN: 1-59120-143-8

Printed in the United States of America

10 9 8 7 6 5 4 3 2

Contents

Introduction

The use of supplemental forms of medicinal mushrooms has gained tremendous popularity among nutrition-oriented practitioners and consumers over the past decade. Centuries of use by Asian herbalists and doctors, solid scientific research, and growing reports in the popular press all have helped to create an explosion of interest in the health benefits offered by mushroom supplements.

Much of this excitement has been generated by clinical research showing mushroom extracts restoring immune competency and improving outcome for people with a variety of serious illnesses, including cancer, hepatitis, asthma, and other conditions where effective nontoxic treatment options are limited.

However, while the health benefits of mushroom supplements are many, "mushroom supplements" as found in the marketplace refer to a large and chemically diverse group of products, very few of which match the potency of the mushroom remedies used in traditional herbalism or the mushroom supplements used in the clinical research, including the research showing immune benefit for chronic illness. Picking the supplement that matches the potency and quality of the supplements used in the supporting research requires that several key issues about medicinal mushroom supplements be understood. This understanding is important if people are to achieve the health benefits and therapeutic results identified in the clinical research and described in the popular literature.

The first issue to consider is the relationship between manufacturing methods and product quality and potency. According to the world's leading mushroom experts, the method by which a mushroom supplement is manufactured is critically important to creating the potency needed to achieve the health benefits identified in traditional herbalism and the clinical research.

The majority of published scientific literature that I was able to locate on the clinical effects and health benefits of using medicinal mushrooms used supplements prepared with hot-water extraction. This is also consistent with the references on traditional use by East Asian herbalists.

The second issue to review is the importance of understanding the descriptions used on the labels of the many diverse forms of mushroom supplements found in your local health food stores and pharmacies. Understanding product descriptions and how they relate to the potency of a product ties into the first issue of manufacturing methods and product quality, helping you to find the potency you need for the benefit you seek.

Many of the primary active compounds in medicinal mushrooms are well known, and research has established the levels needed for prevention and therapeutic benefit. People should be looking for precise potency information on supplement labels and recommended potency levels for all the mushrooms discussed later in the book.

Finally, I will summarize the most common supplemental medicinal mushrooms and their best clinical uses. The goal of this book is to give you the information you need to be an expert on mushroom supplements when you walk into your local health food store. You will be able to choose the mushroom supplement that conforms to the quality standards identified in the research and achieve the desired health benefits offered by medicinal mushrooms.

1

The Nature of Mushrooms

Fungi are an essential part of a sustainable world. They are involved in the decaying and recycling of matter into the nutrients that animals and plants feed on. Medicinal mushrooms in particular help to purify the environment by decomposing dead trees and plants. For humans, there are approximately 700 species that can be eaten as a nutritious food. And, of course, medicinal mushrooms provide a wide variety of health benefits that can contribute to the prevention and treatment of disease.

What is commonly referred to as a "mushroom" is also called the fruit body. This is the part of the fungus that grows above ground, with the sole purpose of releasing spores (seeds) as part of the reproduction cycle. Some fungi do not produce mushrooms and release their spores without a fruiting body.

The spores of fungi are transported by wind and water to a favorable environment where the spores can germinate and generate a new colony. The new colony begins with the threadlike filaments called "hyphae" that emerge from the germinated spores. The original hyphae continue to grow, seeking another compatible hyphae to mate with. After mating, the hyphae branch out in all directions, colonizing the surrounding soil or decaying tree. This weblike collection of interconnected hyphae is then referred to as the "mycelium."

Mycelium lives year round, expanding and growing beneath the surface of the soil or tree. Mycelium works to acquire food, breaking down organic substances in the surrounding soil and decaying wood. It is tightly packed mycelium that actually

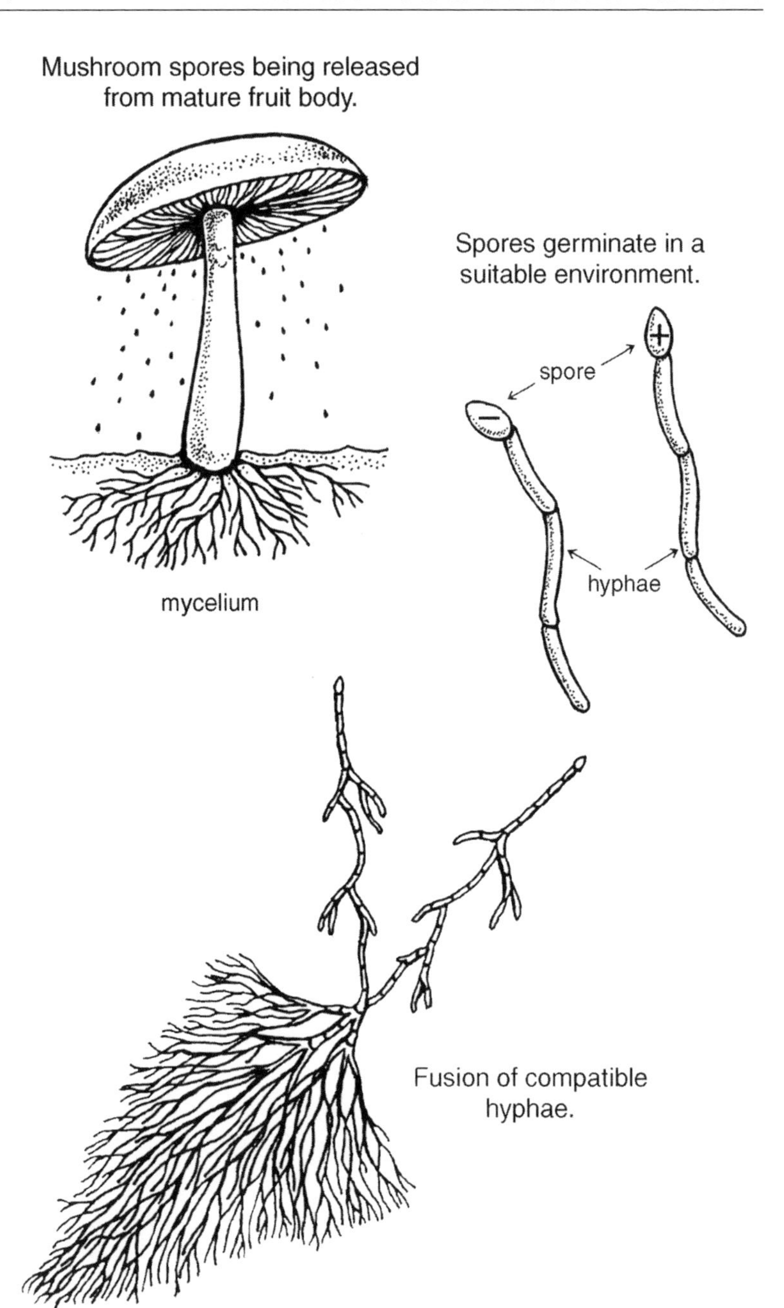

Lifecycle of Mushrooms

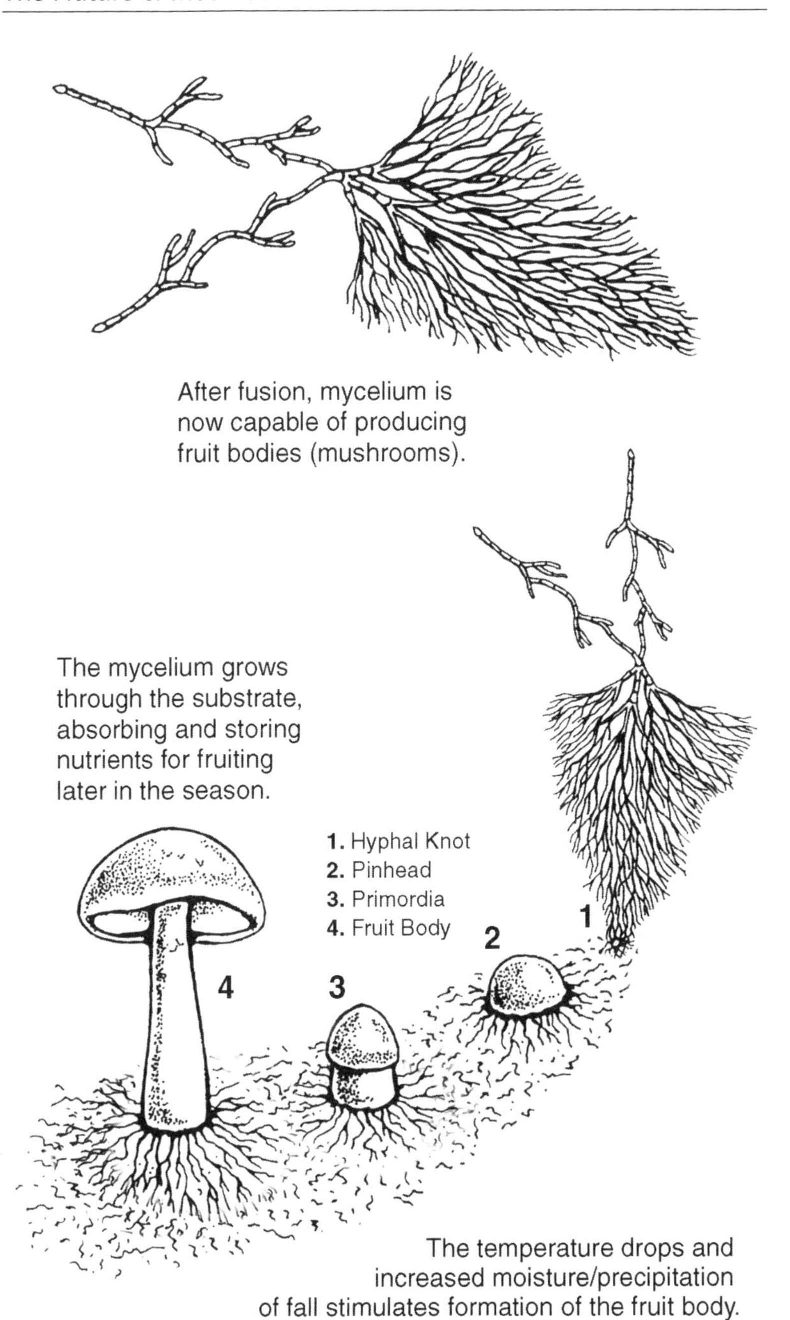

The temperature drops and
increased moisture/precipitation
of fall stimulates formation of the fruit body.

forms the fruit body/mushroom we see above the ground or on tree trunks, typically during spring or fall after the seasonal rain and temperature changes.

Fungi live near the bottom of the ladder in the ecosystem. Similar to humans they have an immune system to protect against a variety of pathogens. During the mycelial stage, when fungi actively digest food and fight hostile competitors, they excrete digestive enzymes to decompose matter. Before the digested food can be absorbed into the cells where the food is used, the fungi must deactivate pathogens and toxins. This is done by releasing special polysaccharides and other disease-fighting chemicals inside the cell walls where the food passes through. This process is believed to provide many of the nutrients that are also invaluable for the human immune system.

Product Quality and Potency

There appears to be a lot of confusion regarding what standards are essential for a therapeutic "mushroom extract." I feel the best way to address this topic is to review how medicinal mushrooms have been used historically and to examine the published scientific data. Traditional Chinese medicine and the medical research represent nearly our entire experience with medicinal mushrooms. Using these two benchmarks, we found a single theme bridging the gap between centuries of historical use as observed in Chinese medicine and the modern experience of validation through scientific research. This common link is hot-water extraction.

Traditional Use

The traditional use of medicinal mushrooms in Chinese medicine and the herbalism of other cultures is very clear. Mushrooms have always been prepared for medicinal use by hot-water extraction. The extraction was done using heat and water in the process of making teas or decoctions. In a decoction, the herb or mushroom is simmered or boiled in water for a period of time, usually 20 to 120 minutes. This should not be confused with an infusion, where water is poured over the herb. Any practitioner of Oriental medicine will verify that decocting is the historical and current method of preparing medicinal mushrooms for tonic use or immune benefit.

Modern Research

A review of the published scientific literature on medicinal mushrooms demonstrates that the majority of mushroom supplements tested in the medical research were hot-water or hot-water/alcohol extracts. This method is used for the most commonly used mushroom extracts, including coriolus, shiitake, maitake, cordyceps, and reishi. Hot-water extraction is also used for all of the well-known isolate products such as Lentinan and LEM from shiitake, Maitake D-Fraction and MaitakeGold 404® from maitake, and PSK/VPS and PSP from *Coriolus versicolor*.

Breaking Down Cell Walls

Many of the rules for preparing plant-based herbs do not apply to mushroom supplements because mushrooms have a unique structure that is completely different from plants. The cell wall in plants is composed of cellulose while mushrooms have a cell wall made of chitin. Chitin is the same hard fiber contained in the shell of a lobster. This is important since chitin is indigestible by humans; yet chitin contains the potent immune-stimulating compounds common to all medicinal mushrooms, the beta-glucans, specific types of polysaccharides. Hot-water extraction is the only proven method for breaking down the chitinous cell walls and releasing the bioactive polysaccharide structurally intact and undamaged. Also, only a heated liquid solution can concentrate the active compounds into therapeutically effective levels in a bioavailable form. This explains why knowledgeable practitioners of traditional East-Asian medicine and modern clinical researchers and doctors use hot-water extraction to overcome the barrier of indigestible chitin.

Some of the popular literature on medicinal mushrooms has suggested that grinding whole dried mushrooms or mycelium to a powder can break up the indigestible cell walls and "release" the beta-glucans contained inside, allowing for their absorption through the digestive process. However, grinding mushrooms is never recommended in traditional herbalism or the medical research. There are a couple of reasons why this might be the case.

As explained in the next section, many scientists believe that the immune-boosting power of beta-glucans is based on their shape. If the grinding is disruptive enough to break down the cell walls in dried mushrooms or mycelium, it also runs the risk of breaking down the structure and shape of the beta-glucans contained inside. Hot-water extraction, by "melting away" the indigestible chitin that surrounds the beta-glucan, maintains the beta-glucan's original shape and structure.

Also, hot-water extraction allows the indigestible fiber to be removed from the supplement, leaving more room in the capsule for active compounds. Grinding removes nothing, leaving a supplement that may contain primarily indigestible fiber. Capsule for capsule, dehydrated hot-water extracts can be up to thirty times more powerful than mycelium biomass.

The Beta-Glucan Connection

The beta-glucans found inside the cell walls of medicinal mushrooms are a specific type of polysaccharide, and, on average, are far more complex than the molecules found in plants. Unlike plant-based molecules, which provide the molecular blueprints for 80 percent of pharmaceutical drugs, the complex polysaccharides in medicinal mushrooms are difficult to reproduce synthetically.

Mushroom beta-glucans are often referred to as "long chain" molecules or "macro" molecules. They consist of multiple spiraling chains of repeating molecular patterns. The spirals and the different patterns of linking create the complex three-dimensional shapes that give the molecules their names.

The term "beta-glucan" is a classification based on structural characteristics with particular designations such as beta 1-4 or beta 1-3 further describing the linking pattern in the long chain molecule. The glucose structure of the beta-glucans is formed from six carbon atoms. Each of the six carbon atoms in the glucose structure is a potential starting or ending point for the links that bind these long chain molecules together. Beta 1-3 has links going from the first to the third carbon, beta 1-4 from the first to the fourth.

In the 1980s, researchers at Harvard University began to understand how critically important shape and structure were to the immune-boosting power of the beta-glucan molecule. Researchers observed a beta-glucan molecule "linking up" with receptors on the surface of an important immune cell, a macrophage. They observed a classic "lock and key" receptor relationship where the shape of the "key," the beta-glucan structure, is all important. This process was observed to stimulate the macrophage activity and soon after, continued research found other examples.

Receptor sites were found on other immune cells such as natural killer cells and neutrophils, and continued research found that different shaped beta-glucans produced different immune responses, immune responses that dramatically improved outcome for a number of serious medical conditions and diseases.

Are All Mushroom Products Equal?

Interestingly, many of the common mushroom supplements prescribed by practitioners or found in health food stores are not manufactured using hot-water extraction. Liquid alcohol tinctures and unextracted forms such as mycelium biomass and dried mushroom powder have little published data on their effectiveness. An informal survey of retail supplement companies that produce or distribute medicinal mushroom products found that few of these companies had published data to support all of their products. This is not to state unconditionally that alcohol tinctures and unextracted products have no value. However, it would make little sense for any trained practitioner or consumer to use a non-hot-water extract when the benefits are unproven and unknown, especially when the clinically proven hot-water extracts are readily available. This is of particular concern as mushroom supplements tend to be used for serious chronic illnesses such as cancer, hepatitis, chronic fatigue, HIV/AIDS, other immune-deficiency conditions, and cardiovascular disease.

In a monograph on Reishi recently published by the American Herbal Pharmacopoeia, the world's top herbal and medical experts on the use of medicinal mushrooms discussed the issues

Mushroom Supplement Descriptions

There are a number of different types of medicinal mushroom supplements and many names to describe them. The following discussion covers most of the descriptions people are likely to find on the labels of mushroom-based supplements.

Mushroom supplements are made from either the mushroom fruit body or the mushroom mycelium. The efficacy of any of these forms of mushroom supplements, as with other supplements, depends on the strength or potency of the preparation. The research indicates that for mushroom supplements, therapeutic strength requires an extraction process that concentrates the active compounds to levels higher than what is found in the unextracted mushrooms or mycelium. Chinese herbal references usually recommend 6 to 20 grams of dried mushrooms daily (or more), prepared as a tea. The research usually recommends 1 to 4 grams of a concentrated hot-water extract daily.

Unextracted Mushroom Supplements

Mycelium Biomass. Mycelium grown on cereal grain that is dried, powdered, and encapsulated. The levels of active compounds are not listed on the label. This material is typically 50 percent undigested grain, by weight.

associated with non-hot water extracts, including the lack of scientific validation, the potential lack of bio-availability, and the low levels of active compounds.

After reviewing the medical research on Reishi they stated that "a review of these data did not appear to be relevant to the use of mycelium products in the United States." The "findings of studies utilizing specific polysaccharides" cannot be used to "substantiate the effectiveness of orally administered com-

Mycelium Powder. Mycelium grown in liquid or on grain that is dried, powdered, and encapsulated. The levels of active compounds are not listed on the label.

"Fruit Body" or "Mushroom" Powder. The mature mushroom fruit body dried, ground to a powder, and encapsulated. Levels of active compounds are not listed on the label.

Extracted Mushroom Supplements

Hydro-Alcohol Extract. It can be made from mycelium grown on grain (mycelium biomass), or the mushroom fruit body. Also know as "tinctures," these liquid "extracts" are preserved in grain or grape alcohol. The levels of active compounds are not listed on the label. Most products state that 30 drops is equal to 1 gram of fresh mushroom or mycelium. As a point of comparison, most herbal sources recommend 6–20 grams of dried mushrooms a day, prepared as a tea. It takes 10 grams fresh to make 1 gram dry.

Hot-Water Extract. Can be made from the mycelium or the mushroom fruit body. Usually the extract is dehydrated into a powder and encapsulated (except Maitake Fractions). With this process the levels of active compounds can be concentrated to specific and desired levels. The levels of active compounds are usually listed on the label as a percentage of total weight.

mercial reishi mushroom mycelium biomass products because of a potential lack of bio-availability. Lastly, most of the studies reviewed used concentrations of isolated constituents that are magnitudes higher than what is available in crude (un-extracted) mycelium biomass preparations."

These experts correctly recognized that the active compounds in unextracted mycelium might still be surrounded by the indigestible chitin. They also acknowledged that the hot-water extraction used to prepare the research supplements created significantly higher levels of active compounds as compared to unextracted supplements.

Although the authors were discussing supplements made from unextracted reishi mycelium, it is important to remember that mushrooms themselves are constructed from tightly packed mycelium. Given the similar structure and shared biology of the medicinal mushrooms and their mycelium, these conclusions likely hold true for all of the non-hot-water extracted mushroom and mycelium supplements.

Nature's Top Seven Medicinal Mushrooms

Medicinal mushrooms are best used based on a person's symptoms and proven clinical uses. In the following chapters, I discuss seven of the most popular medicinal mushrooms and more detailed information on how they work as well as what symptoms/conditions they are most helpful for.

2

Agaricus blazei

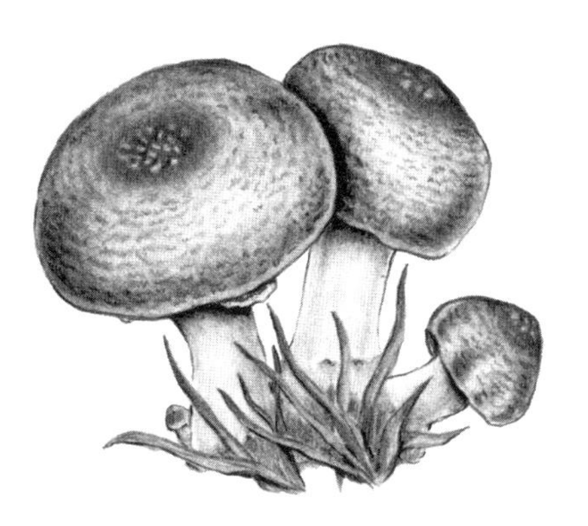

Unlike the other mushrooms covered in this book, *A. blazei* was never used in East Asian herbalism. Instead, it has an extensive history of use as a folk remedy in Brazil. Because this mushroom was heralded by villagers as a longevity tonic, researchers were spurred to take a closer look. This species contains a unique beta-glucan complex that appears to activate many components of the immune system including T lymphocytes, granulocytes, and C3 complement. Animal studies have demonstrated anticancer and antitumor properties. One study also found that *A. blazei* induced apoptosis (self destruction) of malignant cells.

A. blazei has also generated considerable excitement, as some scientists believe it contains the highest levels of beta-glucans among medicinal mushrooms. Although animal and in vitro studies are quite positive, there is a need for more human data.

Supplement Facts	
Amount Per Capsule	
Agaricus blazei fruit body extract 40% Beta Glucan (polysaccharide)	400 mg*
*Daily Value not established	

Minimum potency to look for in *Agaricus blazei*.

Known active constituents: polysaccharides, ergosterols

Clinical Use: Immune modulation, especially in regards to cancer.

Dosage: 1,600–3,200 mg of hot-water extract daily, containing a minimum of 40% polysaccharide (beta-glucan). Take two to four 400-milligram capsules twice daily on an empty stomach.

Safety Profile: Polysaccharides from *A. blazei* are considered nontoxic and safe. As an immune modulator it should be used with extreme care or avoided in organ-transplant patients using immunosuppressive agents.

3

Cordyceps sinensis

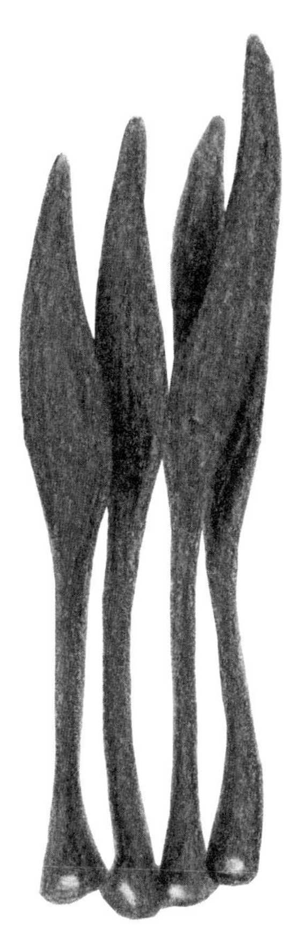

Cordyceps sinensis is also called the "caterpillar fungus," as it grows on and acquires nutrients from several species of caterpillars. In China, it is referred to as "winter worm, summer grass." This fungus is found at high altitude in the mountains of China, Nepal, and Tibet.

Cordyceps attracted the attention of the general public and the health profession in 1993 when a group of Chinese runners broke nine world records in the World Outdoor Track and Field Championships in Germany. The coach of these Chinese athletes attributed those results to the athletes regular use of a *Cordyceps*-based tonic. Because *Cordyceps* helps increase stamina, energy levels, and endurance, it has become one of the top-selling sports supplements among the worlds' elite competitive athletes.

In traditional Chinese medicine, *C. sinensis* is considered to benefit the lung and kidney channels. It is commonly used with the elderly in China as a type of "super-ginseng" for rejuvenation and stamina.

Since it is difficult to collect enough *Cordyceps* from the wild, commercial fermentation methods have been developed in China. These methods are now used here in the West to produce it commercially. Cs-4 is an isolated strain of wild *Cordyceps* that has been the focus of much study and is used by clinics throughout China, and recently in the United States.

Important Studies

Cordyceps has several important uses. The following are conditions for which it has been shown effective in studies.

Improves Fatigue

More than 2,000 patients with a variety of medical problems have been involved with clinical trials of Cs-4 extract. Placebo-controlled studies have found *Cordyceps* to benefit elderly patients with fatigue. Subjective improvements included reduced fatigue, cold intolerance, dizziness, nighttime urination, tinnitus, hyposexuality, and amnesia.

Animal studies suggest that *Cordyceps* improves the ability of organs and tissues to use oxygen more efficiently and increases the production of adenosine triphosphate (ATP) for energy.

Adrenal and Sexual Function

Studies have shown *Cordyceps* to have a homeostatic or balancing effect on adrenal hormones and to protect against adrenal atrophy. Many holistic doctors prescribe *Cordyceps* for supporting and regenerating adrenal gland function.

Along the same lines, human studies have demonstrated benefit in patients reporting low libido. For example, in a double-blind, placebo-controlled, clinical trial, patients who reported decreased sex drives were treated with *Cordyceps.* Those receiving the *Cordyceps* had a subjective improvement rate that was significantly higher than those receiving the placebo. Also, the group receiving *Cordyceps* had a much higher increase in 17-keto-steroid in the urine in a twenty-four-hour period (signifying adrenal stimulation) as compared to those who were receiving placebo. *Cordyceps* has been used in traditional Chinese medicine for the treatment of sexual dysfunction and male impotence.

Respiratory Support

Cordyceps also has a long history of use in the natural treatment of chronic respiratory disorders such as asthma, chronic bronchitis, and other respiratory diseases. Various studies have demonstrated positive effects to improve respiratory function. It should be noted that it takes five to six weeks for asthmatics to see improvement, and the benefits require continued use of the supplement. However, cordyceps can be used for long periods of time without a problem.

Kidney Health

This remarkable fungus has been relied upon by physicians in China for benefit in the treatment of chronic kidney diseases such as chronic nephritis, kidney failure, chronic pyelonephritis, and others. Studies also show that it has a protective effect against chemicals toxic to the kidneys. For example, one study of thirty patients with chronic renal failure found treatment with *Cordyceps* resulted in an overall significant improvement in kidney function. A significant increase in creatinine clearance and a significant reduction in BUN (the concentration of nitrogen in the form of urea in the blood) were noted. In addition, there were significant improvements in anemia, with increases in hemoglobin and red blood cell counts.

Cardiovascular Benefits

Human and animal studies have demonstrated a diverse amount of benefits from *Cordyceps* for the cardiovascular system. This includes positive studies regarding its effects on arrhythmias, ischemic heart disease, and chronic heart failure.

Animal and human studies have shown *Cordyceps* to lower total cholesterol, triglycerides, LDL-C, and VLDL-C, and increased HDL-C. A double-blind, randomized, placebo-controlled study, which lasted two months, looked at the effects of *Cordyceps* on elevated cholesterol levels. Over half of the patients on *Cordyceps* therapy had greater than a 10 percent decrease in total cholesterol and more than a 20 percent decrease in triglycerides, while 76 percent of patients had greater than a 10 percent increase in HDL cholesterol.

Interestingly, animal studies have demonstrated that *Cordyceps* can dilate the coronary arteries and increase blood flow to the heart. This circulatory effect has been shown to also occur with the cerebrovascular arteries and blood supply to the brain.

Other Studies

Smaller studies have also shown *Cordyceps* to have potential value in the treatment of hepatitis B and diabetes.

Cordyceps also has a diverse effect on the immune system. It has been studied in combination with chemotherapy and radiation treatment for lung cancer and patients showed improved tolerance of these therapies with the supplementation of *Cordyceps.*

Supplement Facts	
Amount Per Capsule	
Cordyceps sinensis Cs-4 mycelium extract 14% Beta Glucan (polysaccharide), 6% cordycepic acid, .15% adenosine	400 mg*
*Daily Value not established	

Minimum potency to look for in *Cordyceps sinensis.*

Known active constituents: cordycepin, d-mannitol, adenosine, various polysaccharides

Clinical Use: adrenal fatigue, asthma, athlete's foot, cancer, chronic bronchitis, chronic fatigue, chronic renal failure, decreased libido, diabetes, emphysema, heart disease, hepatitis B, hypercholesterolemia, and tinnitus.

Dosage: 800 to 2,400 milligrams of a hot-water/ethanol extract from fermented mycelia of *Cordyceps sinensis,* strain Cs-4, containing a minimum of 14% polysaccharide (beta-glucan), 6% cordycepic acid, and 0.15% adenosine. Take one to three 400-mg capsules twice daily on an empty stomach.

Safety Profile: Extremely safe. As an immune modulator it should be used with extreme care or even avoided in organ transplant patients using immunosuppressive agents.

4

Coriolus versicolor
(Trametes versicolor)

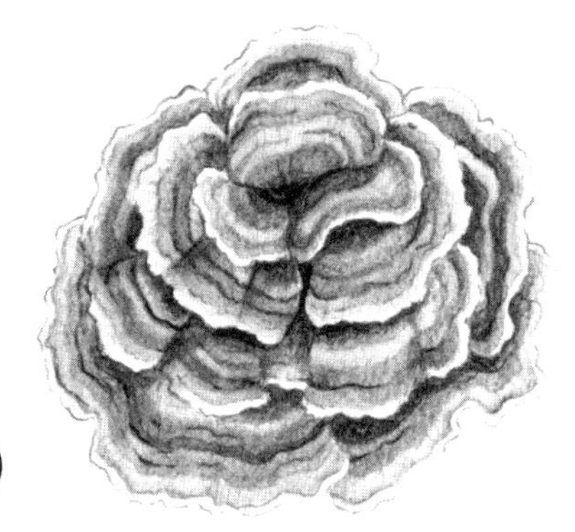

The most well-studied mushroom extract in the world is without a doubt *Coriolus versicolor*. One of the world's leading anticancer drugs was derived from this mushroom.

More than 400 studies have been published that demonstrate the significant immuno-modulating properties of *C. versicolor* in both healthy people and those affected by chronic conditions. *C. versicolor* is very well known in East Asian medicine, especially in the countries of Japan and China. It has an extensive history of use in both traditional and modern conventional practice.

C. versicolor is found in the United States and throughout the temperate forests of the world. It readily grows on logs or on the injured wood of most kinds of trees. It has woody, fruiting bodies that overlap each other and are found on the sides of stumps and tree trunks. *Coriolus* has a unique, plush, velvety surface that is colored in varying shades of brown or gray, with a distinctive pattern of alternating bands of dark and light color. In the West *Coriolus* is referred to as "turkey tail," due to its fan shaped, multicolored cap. *C. versicolor* is also known as *Trametes versicolor*. The Latin translation of *Trametes* is: "one who is thin" and *versicolor* means "variously colored." In Japan it is called Kawaratake, "the mushroom by the river bank," and in China it is referred to as Yun Zhi, meaning "cloud mushroom." In Japan *Coriolus* has been a folk remedy for cancer and in traditional Chinese medicine it is used to dispel phlegm, and to treat pulmonary infections, hepatitis, and cancer.

Origins

Like many of the mushroom extracts, *Coriolus* has an interesting history with respect to its modern applications. In 1965, a chemical engineer for a pharmaceutical company observed his neighbor with late-stage stomach cancer treating himself with *Coriolus.* The engineer convinced his coworkers to study the mushroom. They eventually developed an extract from the mushroom known as PSK, the abbreviation for Polysaccharide-K. The K stands for the first letter of Kureha Chemical, the company that developed PSK, also known as the anticancer drug Krestin. Krestin went on to become a top-selling cancer drug in Japan. This inspired Chinese researchers to develop their own extract. This was accomplished and it is called PSP, an abbreviation for Polysaccharide-peptide. PSP is slightly different from PSK/VPS. PSP has peptide linked beta-glucans, while PSK/VPS have protein linked by beta-glucans.

Chemistry Profile

Protein-bound polysaccharides are the main focus of *Coriolus.* The main component is a beta-D-glucan. The main chain consists of a 1–4 (beta-glucan, with [1,3] beta-glucan and [1,6] beta-glucan) linkages present in smaller amounts. The bioactive protein-bound polysaccharides are found in both the fruiting body and in the mycelium.

Biological Activity

Like other mushroom extracts, *Coriolus* requires a hot-water extraction process to pull the polysaccharides out of the indigestible cell walls. The beta-glucans act as "biological response modifiers" in that they activate many components of the immune system. It has been shown that these beta-glucans pass through the gut wall unchanged and into the bloodstream. Receptors for these beta-glucans have been found on neutrophils, monocytes/macrophages, natural killer cells, and also T and B lymphocytes. Recent American research has also demonstrated significant immuno-modulating activity. These unique polysaccharides have been shown to act as potent inducers of proliferation, tumor cytotoxicity, and lymphokine production by human lymphocytes via in vitro studies.

Clinical Studies

Both PSK and PSP are routinely prescribed in Japan and China to stimulate immune function for people who have had surgical treatment for cancer. It is also widely used for immune support for those undergoing chemotherapy or radiation. It is most commonly prescribed for those undergoing treatment for esophageal, lung, stomach, colon, and breast cancer.

Nonsmall Cell Lung Cancer Stages I–III

In a ten-year study researchers examined the effectiveness of *Coriolus* polysaccharides (PSK) in protecting and promoting immune function in 185 people with lung cancer receiving radiation. The study found that "as a result of administering PSK as adjuvant treatment to patients with epidermoid carcinoma of the lung showing satisfactory tumor shrinkage after radiotherapy, the five-year survival rate of the patients with stages I or II disease, as well as stage III, was 39 percent and 22 percent respectively, compared with the nonadministered group's 16 percent and 5 percent. These differences are statistically significant." In addition, patients aged seventy or older who received the combination of PSK and radiation had a significantly higher survival rate than those who only received radiation.

Coriolus Enhances Disease-Free Period after Colon-Cancer Surgery

A ten-year, randomized, double-blind trial was performed by administering *Coriolus* (PSK) to fifty-six patients and a placebo to another group of fifty-five patients after surgical operations on their colorectal cancers. The rate of patients in remission (or disease free) was significantly higher (more than doubled) in the coriolus group as compared to the placebo group. Researchers also found the white blood cells showed "remarkable enhancement in their activities."

Coriolus Polysaccharides Provide Nutritional Support with Chemotherapy

A 1994 study published in the *Lancet* examined the effect of *Coriolus* polysaccharides (PSK) when added to standard chemotherapy with patients who had undergone curative gastrectomy. Two hundred sixty-two patients were randomly assigned standard treatment alone or with *Coriolus* polysaccharides. The minimum follow-up time was five years. The survival rate of the group using the combination of *Coriolus* polysaccharides and chemotherapy was 73 percent after five years. The group receiving chemotherapy alone had a survival rate of 60 percent. Researchers Hiroaki Nakazato et al., concluded that PSK had "a restorative effect in patients who had been immunosuppressed by both recent surgery and subsequent chemotherapy."

Coriolus Alleviates Side Effects of Chemotherapy and Radiation

A study at the Shanghai Teaching University examined whether *Coriolus* polysaccharides (PSP) could lessen the side effects of chemotherapy or radiation. In this study, 650 people with cancer who were undergoing chemotherapy and radiation were given either PSP or a placebo and their side effects assessed. Researchers used twenty different criteria to assess adverse reactions and determined that those receiving PSP had markedly fewer side effects than those receiving placebo.

Supplement Facts	
Amount Per Capsule	
Coriolus versicolor fruit body extract 20% Beta Glucan (polysaccharide)	400 mg*
*Daily Value not established	

Minimum potency to look for in *Coriolus versicolor.*

Known active constituents: protein-bound polysaccharides (beta-1,4-glucan as the main chain with beta-1,3 glucan and beta-1,6 linkages and amino acids)

Clinical Use: Adjunctive treatment for esophageal, lung, stomach, breast, and colon cancer. Used to prevent side effects and immune suppression from chemotherapy and radiation treatments. Used for infections (of the respiratory, urinary, and digestive tracts), hepatitis B and other liver ailments, HIV, general immune weakness, and ringworm.

Dosage: 1,000–4,000 milligrams daily of a hot-water extract containing a minimum of 20–36% polysaccharide (beta-glucan). Take one to four 400-mg capsules twice daily, morning and evening, on an empty stomach.

Safety Profile: Regarded as extremely safe. As an immune modulator it should be used with extreme care or avoided in organ transplant patients using immunosuppressive agents.

5

Maitake

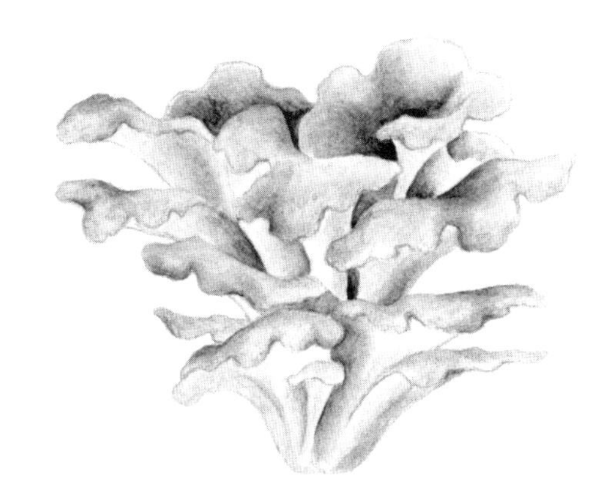

Maitake is one of the best studied mushroom extracts. Indigenous to Northern Japan, maitake has a long history as a valued mushroom, both as a food and as a medicine. Maitake is translated in Japanese as "dancing mushroom." Historical accounts explain the origin of the name, as people would dance with joy when they found maitake because it was so valuable and costly or because maitake is so delicious and healthful. Another explanation is that the fruiting bodies of clustered maitake overlap one another and resemble butterflies in a wild dance.

The Japanese have long used maitake as an adaptogen, a nutrient that helps to balance the various systems and functions of the body.

Evolution of Maitake

In the early 1980s, Dr. Hiroaki Nanba, a professor of microbiology and an expert mycologist at Kobe Pharmaceutical University, was intensively studying the medicinal properties of various mushrooms. During this time, much of his attention was devoted to the popular shiitake mushroom. However, his research showed him that maitake had a unique molecular structure that exhibited greater antitumor activity than other mushroom extracts he had been working with. Maitake, he discovered, also was unique when given orally. In 1984, Dr. Nanba discovered an important maitake fraction (or specialized component) that stimulated macrophages. Through a special extraction method, these maitake fractions were isolated. It was now possible to produce a standardized form of specific beta-glucan polysaccharides—beta-1,6 glucan and beta-1,3 glucan. Later in his research, Dr. Nanba patented what is known as MaitakeGold 404®.

According to studies, maitake fractions have the ability to both directly enhance the damaging activity of NK cells against cancer cells and to change NK precursor cells into activated NK cells.

Immune Properties of Maitake

Dr. Nanba and other researchers have identified several mechanisms through which maitake beta-glucans provide immune support. Several Japanese studies have been published regarding the immuno-modulating effects of maitake.

In 1998, researchers at the University of Massachusetts at Amherst found that an extract of maitake had significant inhibitory activity against human cervical cancer and T4 leukemic cells. The researchers concluded that further studies were definitely warranted.

Reduces Chemotherapy Side Effects

Maitake is becoming popular to help reduce the side effects of chemotherapy. A survey of 671 patients showed that combining chemotherapy with maitake treatment can reduce adverse reactions (such as hair loss, pain, and nausea) as well as diminish the pain that comes with terminal stage cancer.

Maitake also appears to make chemotherapy more effective. One study compared the effects of maitake beta-glucan extract and the chemotherapy drug mitomycin (MMC) on mice with cancer. The maitake beta-glucan alone inhibited tumor growth more effectively (80 percent) than MMC alone (45 percent). However, the most effective tumor inhibition was observed with the combination of these two substances with almost 98 percent inhibition. This is an interesting partnership as maitake supports immune function while the MMC directly kills tumor cells.

Cancer Study

A total of thirty-three cancer patients in stages II, III, and IV, ages thirty-three to sixty-eight, participated in this trial. Data was collected under the cooperation of their medical doctors in Japan. Patients were given either maitake beta-glucan with tablets only, or maitake beta-glucan and tablets in addition to chemotherapy. Cancer regression or significant symptom improvement was observed in eleven out of sixteen breast cancer patients, seven out of twelve liver cancer patients, and five out of eight lung cancer patients.

Maitake appears to be most effective against breast, prostate, and liver cancers. To date, it has been less effective against bone, blood, and brain cancers.

Supplement Facts

Amount Per Capsule	
Grifola frondosa (Maitake) fruit body extract 20% Beta Glucan (polysaccharide)	400 mg*

*Daily Value not established

Minimum potency to look for in maitake.

Known active constituents: beta-1,3 glucan and beta-1,6 glucan

Clinical Use: Adjunctive cancer treatment, fatigue, high blood pressure, liver disease, and HIV, antioxidant.

Dosage: 300–2,400 mg of a hot-water extract daily, containing a minimum of 20% polysaccharide (beta-glucan). Take one to four capsules twice daily, morning and evening, on an empty stomach. Maitake fractions dosage: for immune support, take 0.5 to 1 milligram of MaitakeGold 404 per kilogram (2.2 pounds) of body weight per day.

Safety Profile: Extremely safe. As an immune modulator it should be used with extreme care or avoided in organ transplant patients using immunosuppressive agents.

6

Reishi

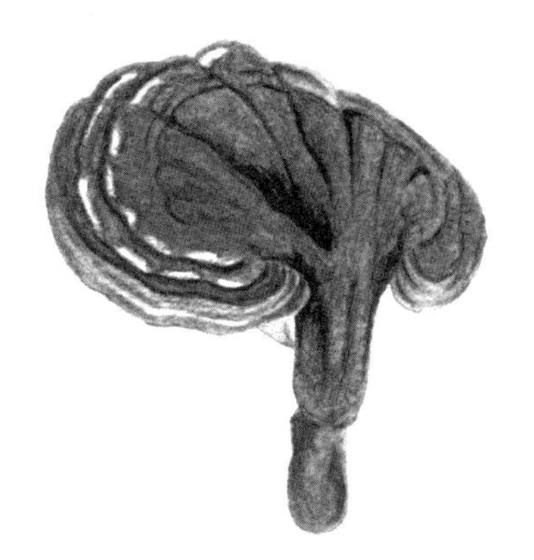

The reishi mushroom (*Ganoderma lucidum*) is one of the most revered herbs in traditional Chinese and Japanese medicine, with a documented history of over 2,000 years. Known as Ling Zhi in China, there are references to its use in that country as far back as 100 B.C. where it was referred to as the "Herb of Spiritual Potency" and the "Ten-Thousand-Year Mushroom."

Reishi is one of the most highly regarded medicinal mushrooms and is probably the best choice when looking for a general health tonic to improve overall health and increase longevity. It is considered an adaptogen.

Modern clinical research also supports many of the uses for this mushroom as described in traditional medicine. It benefits immune health, cardiovascular health, and liver function. Reishi is also frequently used by mountain climbers to combat altitude sickness and is contained in many of the performance-enhancing herbal formulas used by Chinese athletes.

The fruiting bodies of reishi range from a reddish-orange to an almost black color. The fruiting body also has a shiny look to it (*lucidum* translates to "shiny"). Reishi is extremely difficult to find in the wild but is successfully cultivated for commercial purposes.

Research has demonstrated that reishi has several different active constituents. One group of active constituents is the polysaccharides. The various types of polysaccharides found in reishi have demonstrated immune-enhancing properties. This includes enhancement of several important interleukins.

Another major class of compounds is the triterpenes. These compounds have been reported to have adaptogenic, anti-hypertensive, and anti-allergy effects. Many of the important triterpenes are found only in the mushroom. They are extracted from the shiny red surface of the mushroom, a physical feature missing in the mycelium.

Cardiovascular Benefits

Reishi has been shown in some studies to inhibit platelet aggregation and reduce blood pressure. In one study of thirty-three people with hypertension researchers found blood pressure was significantly reduced over two-weeks' time with reishi supplementation.

Reishi is currently being used in Chinese medicine for the treatment of hypercholesterolemia. It appears to reduce cholesterol via two mechanisms. One is the inhibition of endogenous cholesterol synthesis by inhibiting HMG-CoA Reductase and by inhibiting cholesterol absorption from food sources.

Immune Benefits

Reishi is commonly prescribed by practitioners for long-term immune system support. This includes its use as an adjunctive therapy for cancer. For example, in one placebo-controlled study, forty-eight patients with advanced tumors were given reishi mushroom extract for thirty days. Researchers found a marked immune-modulating effect as demonstrated by an increase in T lymphocytes and decreased CD8 counts. Patients also reported reduced side effects due to chemotherapy or radiation as well as postoperation recovery.

Several studies have demonstrated antitumor activity in animals. More studies are required to confirm this activity in humans.

Studies in China have demonstrated a substantial improvement for patients with chronic bronchitis. In a study of over 2,000 patients with chronic bronchitis there was a 60 to 90 percent improvement within two weeks after beginning a reishi syrup.

Blood Sugar Balance

Animal and in vitro studies have shown reishi to have a blood sugar lowering effect. Much of this activity appears to be due to polysaccharides known as Ganoderans A, B, and C.

It appears there are three main mechanisms behind this hypoglycemic effect. This includes Reishi's ability to elevate plasma insulin levels, to enhance peripheral tissue utilization of glucose, and to enhance liver metabolism of glucose.

Anti-inflammatory Effects

Various animal and in vitro studies have shown that hot-water/ethanol extracts of reishi have anti-inflammatory effects. One study found that 220 milligrams of reishi extract and 50 milligrams of reishi powder had comparable effects to 5 milligrams of hydrocortisone.

Liver Protector

Reishi is commonly used for its hepatoprotective (liver protective) action. One small study of four patients with hepatitis B and elevated liver enzymes (SGOT/SGPT) and bilirubin were given 6 grams of reishi for three months. Significant reduction in SGOT and SGPT were noticed within one month. After three months all values were within normal range.

Altitude Sickness

One of the unique uses of reishi is for altitude sickness. Reishi appears to reduce altitude sickness by oxygenating the blood. This benefit was studied in Chinese mountain climbers that ascended mountains as high as 17,000 feet with minimal reaction. Daily use of reishi should be started ten to fourteen days before you climb the mountain.

Known active constituents: polysaccharides, triterpenes (Ganoderic acids), ergosterols

Clinical Use: Daily tonic to improve and maintain good health, long-term immune support, hepatitis C, hypercholesterolemia, altitude sickness, and diabetes.

Supplement Facts	
Amount Per Capsule	
Ganoderma lucidum (Red Reishi), fruit body extract, 10% Beta Glucan (polysaccharide), 4% Triterpenes (ganoderic acids)	400 mg*
*Daily Value not established	

Minimum potency to look for in reishi.

Dosage: 800 to 4,000 milligrams per day of a hot-water/ethanol extract, containing a minimum of 10% polysaccharide (beta-glucan) and 4% triterpene. Take one to five 400-mg capsules twice daily, morning and evening, on an empty stomach.

Decoction: 375 milliliters twice daily

Safety Profile: No toxicity reported. Occasional digestive upset or skin rash in sensitive users. Caution is advised for those currently using blood-thinning medications due to reishi's anticoagulant effects. Also, caution is advised for those taking hypoglycemic medication due to reishi's potential hypoglycemic activity. As an immune modulator it should be used with extreme care or avoided in organ transplant patients using immunosuppressive agents.

7

Shiitake

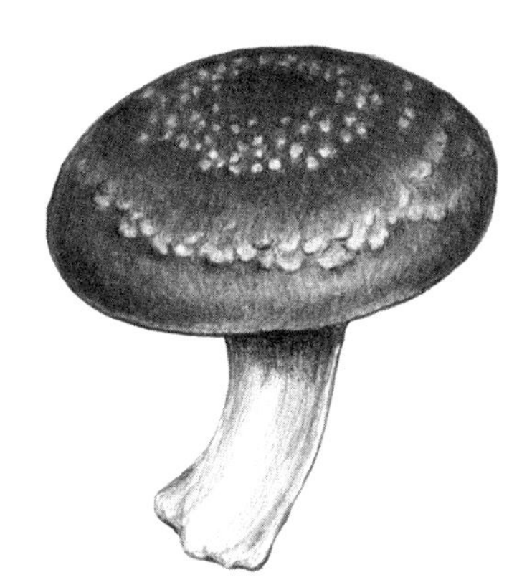

Shiitake (*Lentinula Edodes*) is regarded as a gourmet food in the West, while in Japan and China shiitake is known to be a valuable food and medicinal agent. Its name comes from the Japanese chestnut tree, *shiia,* and the Japanese word for mushroom, *take.* It is also referred to as the "fragrant mushroom" or the "forest mushroom."

This mushroom is indigenous to Japan, China, and other areas of Asia. It is not found in the wild in America but is cultivated for commercial use. Shiitake is the second most common edible mushroom in the world. The fungi is found on dead and injured hardwood trees, including the chestnut tree, hence the prefix *shiia.* Shiitake has a medicinal history of more than 1,000 years and was revered by Japanese emperors. It has been used in traditional Chinese medicine to treat colds, flu, and cardiovascular disease.

Shiitake is used medicinally in two forms in Asia and around the world. This includes lentinan, a purified polysaccharide extracted from the cell wall of the Shiitake fruiting body. The second extract is known as Lentinula edodes mycelium extract, better known as LEM. Both extracts have been shown to enhance immune activity. Both forms have been shown to have a beneficial effect orally but the majority of published data on lentinan has been with the injectable or intravenous forms.

Adjuvant Cancer Therapy

As with many of the medicinal mushrooms, Shiitake has been shown to be of benefit as an adjuvant cancer therapy. It has been shown to improve specific immune markers (including natural killer cells, tumor necrosis factor, T-helper cells, and a variety of interleukins), and patient outcomes. For example, in a study of sixteen people with advanced cancer, lentinan was injected into areas of malignancy. Researchers found that 80 percent of the lesions showed a clinical response, and the survival time for those patients who responded was 129 days and 49 days for those who did not respond.

In a randomized, controlled trial, 275 people with advanced or recurrent stomach cancer were given either chemotherapy and lentinan injections or chemotherapy alone. Using a variety of parameters for analysis, researchers found that the best results occurred when lentinan was given prior to chemotherapy.

Infections

Shiitake extracts have demonstrated a wide variety of activity against various microbes. This includes bacteria (including *Mycobacterium tuberculosis*), parasites, and viruses (including HIV and hepatitis B). More human data is needed to corroborate these initial findings, which were mainly from animal studies.

Cardiovascular Benefits

Current research is demonstrating that shiitake extracts are a promising treatment for high cholesterol levels and for high blood pressure. Human studies have shown that the consumption of high amounts of fresh and dried shiitake resulted in cholesterol decreases that ranged from 7 to 14 percent.

Supplement Facts	
Amount Per Capsule	
Lentinula edodes (Shiitake) extract 10% Beta Glucan (polysaccharide)	400 mg*
*Daily Value not established	

Minimum potency to look for in shiitake.

Known active constituents: polysaccharides with 1-3 beta-D-glucan linkages and a special beta-1,6-D-glucopyranoside branching

Clinical Use: Immune-suppressive diseases such as HIV/AIDS, cancer, colds, flus, candidiasis, high cholesterol, and hepatitis.

Dosage: 800 to 3,000 milligrams of a hot-water extract daily, containing a minimum of 10–20% polysaccharide (beta-glucan). Take one to five capsules twice daily, morning and evening, on an empty stomach.

Safety Profile: Shiitake and the extracts lentinan and LEM are considered nontoxic. There are reports in the literature of rare sensitivity reactions that result in dermatitis.

8

Hericium erinaceus

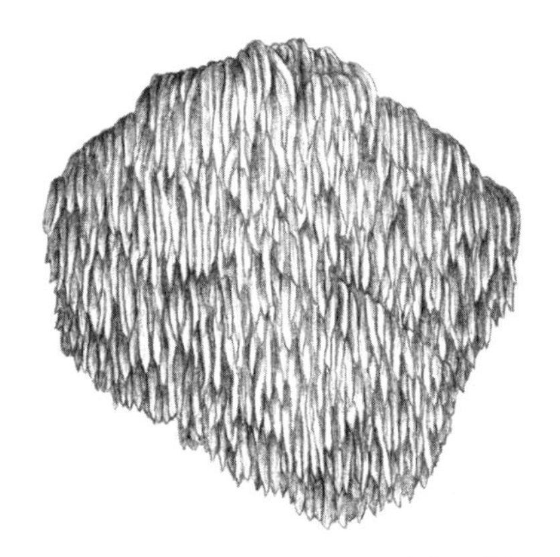

The most recent mushroom extract to excite natural-health enthusiasts is *Hericium erinaceus*. Because it resembles white, icelike pillars, a host of names have arisen to describe it, such as Lion's Mane, Monkey's Head, Monkey's Mushroom, Bear's Head, Old Man's Beard, White Beard, and Hedgehog Mushroom. In Japan it is referred to as Yambushitake and in China it is called Shishigashira. Lion's Mane is found throughout North America, East Asia, and Europe. Besides being used as a medicinal mushroom, Lion's Mane is a choice edible.

Traditional Chinese and Native American Uses

Hericium erinaceus is used in traditional Chinese medicine for the treatment of digestive tract ailments. *H. erinaceus* extract, known as Houtou, is used topically on scratches and cuts to stop bleeding by Native Americans and others.

Immune Properties

H. erinaceus has been the subject of recent studies involving the immune system. As with most of the medicinal mushrooms, unique polysaccharides present in *H. erinaceus* have immune-enhancing properties, and preliminary studies are demonstrating some anticancer effects.

Neurological Properties

The most intriguing potential of *H. erinaceus* is that it may stimulate the production of a substance known as Nerve Growth Factor (NGF). This specialized protein is necessary for the growth of sensory neurons. An in vitro study found that an extract from this mushroom promoted myelin sheath growth on brain cells. The myelin sheath is an important component of neurons that is involved in the transmission of nerve messages. Researchers hope that *H. erinaceus* will prove to be helpful for Alzheimer's disease and other degenerative, neurological conditions. Further studies are needed to clarify whether *H. erinaceus* has any benefit for human neurological conditions.

Supplement Facts	
Amount Per Capsule	
Hericium erinaceus (Lion's Mane) extract 15% Beta Glucan (polysaccharide)	400 mg*
*Daily Value not established	

Minimum potency to look for in *Hericium erinaceus*.

Known active constituents: beta-glucans/polysaccharides, hericenones, erinacines

Safety Profile: No known contraindications or drug interactions.

Clinical Use: Digestive tract ailments, including ulcers and stomach cancer. Cognitive enhancement.

Dosage: 1,000 to 4,000 milligrams of a hot-water extract daily, containing a minimum of 15% polysaccharide (beta-glucan). Take one to five capsules twice daily, morning and evening, on an empty stomach.

9

How to Take Mushroom Supplements

The first step in successfully using mushroom supplements is to understand how to read the label. In general this is best done by reviewing the *Supplement Facts* on the product label. The bottle should clearly state:

1. Mushroom name.
2. Type of extract (look for products that are formulated to the potencies given in the previous mushroom descriptions). This should include the guaranteed percentage and polysaccharide description, unless it is a well-researched isolate, such as MaitakeGold 404.
3. Check with the manufacturer to confirm extraction techniques (hot-water or hot-water/alcohol extracts) as well as quality assurance.

Hot-water extracted mushroom supplements are usually dehydrated and sold as capsules (except maitake fractions). Hot-water extracts also list the levels of active compounds on the label, making it easy to distinguish them from the other less potent forms of mushroom supplements. Take the recommended dosage between meals for optimal results. If you notice minor digestive upset when taking mushroom extracts on an empty stomach try taking the supplement with food.

Conclusion

There are a variety of medicinal mushrooms that can be used to improve one's health. They represent some of the most effective immune-supportive supplements in the natural foods industry. Historical use and published research has consistently shown that hot-water extracts are the preferred method of extraction for most medicinal mushrooms and mycelium in order to attain therapeutic levels of active constituents. It is also important to select the mushroom extract that is most highly recommended for a particular condition for optimal benefits.

Summary of Medicinal Mushroom Uses

Agaricus = antitumor

Cordyceps = lung, kidneys, adrenals, energy, libido, asthma, bronchitis, and tinnitus

Coriolus = chemotherapy support; lung, colon, liver, breast, and stomach cancer; and HIV

Maitake = breast and prostate cancer, and HIV

Reishi = liver, cholesterol, and daily immune tonic; hepatitis; HIV; anti-inflammatory; antiviral

Shiitake = antimicrobial, cholesterol, immune support

Hericium = stomach and cognitive enhancement

References

Alexopoulos, C. J. and C. W. Mims. *Introductory Mycology.* Wiley, 1979, p. 10.

Aoki,T. 1984. "Lentinan." In *Immune Modulation Agents and Their Mechanisms,* R. L. Fenichel and M. A. Chirgis, eds. *Immunology Studies.* 25:62–77.

Bensky, D., et al. *Materia Medica of Chinese Herbal Medicine.* Eastland Press, Seattle, 1993, pp. 338–39.

Chang, H. M. and P. But. *Pharmacology and Applications of Chinese Materia Medica.* Vol.1. Singapore: World Scientific, 1986.

Chen, D. G. Effects of JinShuiBao capsule on the quality of life of patients with chronic heart failure. *J Administration Traditional Chinese Med* 5(suppl), (1995):40–45.

Chen, Y. P., et al. Comparisons of fermented *Cordyceps mycelia* and natural *Cordyceps sinensis* in treating 30 patients with renal failure. *Chinese Traditional Herbal Drugs* 17(6), (1986):256–258.

Cheng, Z., et al. Effects of ling zhi on hemorrheology parameters and symptoms of hypertension patients with hyperlipidemia and sequelae of cerebral thrombosis. In: Shu S. and M. Mori, eds., *The Research on* Ganoderma lucidum (*Part One*). Volume 1. Shanghai Med Univ., 1993, pp. 339–342.

Cheng, J. H., et al. Analysis of therapeutic effect of Jinshuibao capsule in adjuvant treatment of 20 patients with terminal stage of lung cancer. *J Administration Traditional Chinese Med* 5(suppl), (1995): 34–35.

Chihara, G., et al. Inhibition of mouse sarcoma 180 by polysaccharides from *Lentinus edodes* (Shiitake). *Nature,* 222 (1969): 637.

Feng, M. G., et al. Vascular dilation by fermented mycelia of *Cordyceps sinensis* in anesthetized dogs. *J Chinese Materia Medica* 12(12), (1987):745–749.

Fujimaya, Y., et al. Tumor specific cytocidal and immunopotentiating effects of relatively low molecular weight products derived from the basidiomycete, *Agaricus blazei* Murill. *Anticancer Res,* 19 (1999):113–118.

Fujimiya, Y., et al. Selective tumoricidal effect of soluble proteglucan extracted from the basidiomycete, Agaricus blazei Murill, mediated via natural killer cell activation and apoptosis. Cancer Immunol Immunother, 46 (1998):147–159.

Hans, SR. Experiences in treating patients of chronic bronchitis and pulmonary diseases with Cs-4 capsule (JinShuiBao). *J. Administration Traditional Chinese Med* 5(suppl), (1995): 33–34.

Hayakawa, K., N. Mitsuhashi, and Y. Saito, et al. Effect of krestin (PSK) as adjuvant treatment on the prognosis after radical radiotherapy in patients with non-small cell lung cancer. *Anticancer Res.,* 13(5C): September–October, (1993): 1815–1820.

He, X. G., Seleen, J., Chemical Analysis as Quality Control Method for Medicinal Mushroom Extracts, *International Journal of Medicinal Mushrooms,* 6(3), (2004) 253–261.

Hikino, H., et al. Mechanisms of hypoglycemic activity of ganodernan B: A glycan of *Ganoderma lucidum* fruit bodies. *Planta Med* 55(4), (1989):385.

Hiroaki, Nakazato, et al. Efficacy of immunochemotherapy as adjuvant treatment after curative resection of gastric cancer. *Lancet* vol. 343 (1994).

Hobbs, C. *Medicinal Mushrooms.* Loveland, CO: Interweave Press Inc., 1996, p.110.

Huang, Y., et al. Toxicity study of fermentation *Cordyceps mycelia* B1414. Zhongchengyao Yanjiu (10), (1987): 24–25.

Ikuzawa, M., et al. Fate and Distribution of an Anti-Tumor Protein-Bound Polysaccharide PSK (Krestin). *International Journal of Immunopharmacology* 10(4), (1988): 415–423.

Ito, H., et al. Anti-tumor effects of a new polysaccharide-protein complex (ATOM) prepared from *Agaricus blazei* (Iwade strain 101) and its mechanisms in tumor-bearing mice. *Anticancer Res.,* 17 (1997): 277–284.

Jong, S. C. and J. M. Birmingham. Medicinal benefits of the mushroom *Ganoderma. Adv Appl Microbiol* 37 (1992):101–134.

Kolotushkina, E. V., M. G. Moldavan, and K. Y. Voronin, et al. The influence of *Hericium erinaceus* extract on myelination process in vitro. *Fiziol Zh* 49(1), 2003: 38–45.

Kupin, V. A new biological response modifier *Ganoderma lucidum* and its application in oncology. In: Proceedings of the 4th international symposium on *Ganoderma lucidum;* Seoul. Cancer Res Ctr, June 10, 1992, pp.49–50.

Liu, B., and Y. Bau. *Fungi Pharmacopoeia.* Kiniko Press, 1980, pp. 170–172.

Lou, Y., et al. Cardiovascular pharmacological studies of ethanol extracts of *Cordyceps mycelia* and *Cordyceps* fermentation solution. *Chinese Traditional and Herbal Drugs* 17(5), (1986):17–21; 209–213.

Lovy, A., B. Knowles, and R. Labbe, et al. Activity of edible mushrooms against the growth of human T4 leukemic cancer cells, HeLa cervical cancer cells, and Plasmodium falciparum. *Journal of Herbs, Spices, and Medicinal Plants* 6(4), (1998): 49–57.

Manabe, N., et al. Effects of the mycelial extract of cultured *Cordyceps sinensis* on in vivo hepatic energy metabolism in the mouse. *Jpa J Pharmacol* (1), (1996):85–88.

Mizuno, M., et al. Polysaccharides from *Agaricus blazei* stimulate lymphocyte T cell subsets in mice. *Biosoci Biotechnol Biochem.* 62 (1998):434–437.

Morikawa, K., R. Takeda, M.Yamazaki, et al. Induction of tumoricidal activity of polymorphonuclear leukocytes by a linear 1,3-D-glucan and other immuno-modulators in murine cells. *Cancer Res.* 45: (1985): 1496–1501.

Nakazato H., A. Koike, and S. Saji, et al. Efficacy of immunochemotherapy as adjuvant treatment after curative resection of gastric cancer. Study Group of Immunochemotherapy with PSK for Gastric Cancer. *Lancet* 7;343(8906), (May 1994):1122–1126.

Nanba, H. Maitake D fraction: Healing and preventive potential for cancer. *J Orthomol Med* 12(1), 1997: 43–49.

——. *Maitake Challenges Cancer.* Kobe, Japan: Socio Health Group, 1998.

——. Presented at the 3rd International Conference on Mushroom Biology and Mushroom Products in Sydney, Australia (October 1999).

Nanba, H. and P. Kumar. *The Therapeutics of Maitake Mushroom in Japan.* Kobe, Japan: New Editions Health World, 1995, p. 21.

Oka, M., et al. Immunological analysis and clinical effects of intrabdominal and intrapleural injection of lentinan for malignant ascites and pleural effusion. *Biotherapy* 5 (1992):107–112.

Shao, G., et al. Treatment of hyperlipidemia with *Cordyceps sinensis:* A double blind placebo control trial. *Intl J Orient Med* 15(2), (1990): 77–80.

Shiao, M. S., et al. Natural products and biological activities of the Chinese medicinal fungus *Ganoderma lucidum. Am Chem Soc* 547 (1994):342–354.

Soo, T. S. The therapeutic value of *Ganoderma lucidum.* In Buchanan et al., *Ganoderma systematics, phytopathology and pharmacology.* Proceedings of contributed symposium 59A, B; 5th International Mycological Congress; Vancouver (August 14–21, 1994), pp.105–113.

Stavinhoa, W. B., et al. Study of the anti-inflammatory activity of *Ganoderma lucidum.* Research paper presented at the Third Academic/Industry Joint Conference; August 18–20, 1990; Sapporo Park Hotel (Japan).

Sun, Z., et al. The ameliorative effect of PSP on the toxic and side reaction of chemo and radiotherapy of cancers. In *Advanced Research in PSP,* Q. Yang, ed.

Hong Kong: Hong Kong Association for Health Care Ltd., 1999 Suzuki, S. and S. Ohshima. Influence of Shi-Ta-Ke (*Lentinus edodes*) on human serum cholesterol. *Mushroom Science IX (Part 1)*. Proceedings of the Ninth International Scientific Congress on the Cultivation of Edible Fungi, Tokyo (1974): 463–467.

Taguchi, T., et al. 1982. Clinical Trials on Lentinan (Polysaccharide). In Yamamura, Y., et al. (eds.) *Immunomodulation by Microbial Products and Related Synthetic Compounds.* New York: Elsevier Science Publishing Company, pp. 467–475.

Tomada, M., et al. Glycan structures of ganoderans B and C, hypoglycemic glycans of *Ganoderma lucidum* fruit bodies. *Phytochemistry* 25:28 (1988):17–20.

Torisu, M., Y. Hayashi and T. Ishimitsu, et al. Significant prolongation of disease-free period gained by oral polysaccharide K (PSK) administration after curative surgical operation of colorectal cancer. *Cancer Immunol Immunother* 31(5), (1990):261–268.

Torisu, M., et al. Significant prolongation of disease-free period gained by oral PSK (*Coriolus* versicolor) administration after curative surgical operation of colon cancer. *Cancer Immunology Immunotherapy* 31 (1990):261–268.

Upton, R., et al. Reishi Mushroom (*Ganoderma lucidum*) Standards of Analysis, Quality Control, and Therapeutics. *American Herbal Pharmacopoeia* (September 2000), p. 9.

Wang, J.C., S. H. Hu, C. H. Su, et al. Antitumor and immunoenhancing activities of polysaccharide from culture broth of *Hericium* spp. *Fiziol Zh* 49(1), (2003):38–45.

Xie, Z., et al. *Dictionary of Traditional Chinese Medicine.* The Commercial Press Ltd., Hong Kong, (1988), p. 201.

Xu, J. M. and H. J. Zheng. Treating 64 patients with arrhythmia by Ningxinbao capsule: A randomized, double-blind observation. *Shanghia J Traditional Chinese Med* (4):4–5:1994.

Yang, W., et al. Clinical study of fermentation product of *Cordyceps sinensis* on treatment of hyposexuality. *J Admin Traditional Chinese Med* 5(suppl) (1995):23–24.

Zhang, Z., et al. Clinical and laboratory studies of JinShuiBao in cavenging oxygen free radicals in elderly senescent XuZheng patients. *J Admin Traditional Chinese Med* 5 (suppl) 1995:14–18.

Zhou, L. T., et al. Short term curative effect of cultured *Cordyceps sinensis* (Berk) Sacc. Mycelia in chronic hepatitis B. China *J Chinese Materia Medica* 15(1) (1990): 14–18;53–55.

Index

About the Author

Mark Stengler, N.D., is a leading naturopathic doctor and author of more than sixteen books on natural healing. These include the best-selling *The Natural Physician's Healing Therapies and Prescription for Natural Cures*. He is a frequent guest on national television and radio shows. Dr. Stengler served on a committee for the Yale University Complementary Medicine Outcomes Research Project. He is in private practice in La Jolla, California. His website is www.lajollawholehealth.com.